The Miracle Elixir

Unlocking the Secrets and Benefits of Castor Oil

Donald K. Armstrong

Published by Kindle Direct Publishing

Seattle, Washington,

United States

Kdp.amazon.com

Author Profile

Donald K. Armstrong is a seasoned health writer with a passion for translating complex medical information into accessible and engaging content. Armed with a background in health sciences and journalism, Armstrong has dedicated his career to bridging the gap between medical expertise and public understanding.

With a keen interest in promoting wellness and preventive care, Armstrong's writing style combines clarity, accuracy, and a touch of empathy. He has a knack for breaking down intricate medical concepts into digestible pieces, empowering readers to make informed decisions about their health.

Armstrong's work spans various health topics, from fitness and nutrition to mental well-being and chronic disease management. His articles not only provide valuable insights into the latest medical research but also offer practical tips and advice for readers to implement in their everyday lives.

Having contributed to reputable health publications, Armstrong remains committed to delivering reliable and up-to-date information to his audience. His mission is to inspire and educate, fostering a healthier and more informed society through the power of words. Whether addressing the latest health trends or debunking common myths, Donald K. Armstrong is a trusted voice in the realm of health and wellness writing.

Table of Contents

Unveiling the Elegance of Castor Oil in Beauty and Personal Care

- Natural Skincare Recipes
- Castor Oil Cleansing Routine
- DIY Face Masks
- Deep Conditioning
- Scalp Massage Techniques

Risks and Precautions

- Allergic Reactions
- Dosage and Application Guidelines
- Consultation with Healthcare Professionals

Choosing the Right Castor Oil

- Understanding types of castor oil
- Check for purity
- Consider the extraction method
- Assess color and odor
- Packaging matters
- Consider your purpose
- Read customer reviews
- Check for certifications

- Price vs. quality balance

Conclusion

- Recap of Key Benefits
- Incorporating Castor Oil into Your Daily Routine

Introduction

Understanding castor oil

Castor oil is a dense and scentless oil derived from castor plant seeds. Its history traces back to ancient Egypt, where it served various purposes such as a lamp fuel, medicine, and beauty treatment. Cleopatra herself is said to have used it to enhance the whiteness of her eyes.

In modern times, India is the main producer of castor oil. It continues to be utilized as a remedy for constipation and is a common ingredient in skincare and haircare products. Interestingly, it is also found in motor oil. The FDA approves its safety for treating constipation, but ongoing research is exploring potential additional health benefits.

Castor oil isn't meant for eating because it doesn't taste good. However, some folks use a little bit of it for health reasons.

According to MyFitnessPal, one tablespoon of castor oil has:

- Calories: 120

- Protein: 0 grams

- Fat: 14 grams

- Carbohydrates: 0 grams

- Fiber: 0 grams

- Sugar: 0 grams

Castor oil also contains:

- Vitamin E

- Omega-9 fatty acids

- Omega-6 fatty acids

The main ingredient in castor oil that does most of its function is a fatty acid called ricinoleic acid.

Not much study has been done on the traditional health uses of this oil. However, it may have some health advantages, although more research is needed to confirm them.

- **Constipation**

Castor oil is only approved by the FDA for a specific health purpose: to help with occasional constipation as a natural laxative. When you take castor oil, a component called ricinoleic acid interacts with receptors in your intestines. This interaction triggers the muscles in your intestines to contract, assisting in the movement of stool through your colon.

Sometimes, people use castor oil to cleanse the colon before medical procedures like a colonoscopy. However, your doctor may recommend other laxatives that could be more effective.

Avoid using castor oil for prolonged periods to relieve constipation because it may lead to side effects such as cramps and bloating. If you experience constipation for more than a few days, it's important to consult with your doctor.

- **Inducing labor**

For many years, people have used castor oil to assist with childbirth. A study from 1999 revealed that 93% of midwives in the United States used it to start labor. However, research on its effectiveness has produced mixed results, with some studies suggesting benefits and others showing no significant impact. If you're expecting a baby, it's crucial to consult your doctor before considering the use of castor oil during pregnancy.

- **Anti-inflammatory effects**

Studies on animals suggest that ricinoleic acid, when applied to the skin, might be helpful in reducing swelling and pain caused by inflammation. There's even a study in people suggesting it works as well as a common anti-inflammatory drug for treating symptoms of knee arthritis. However, more research is needed to fully understand and confirm these potential benefits.

- **Healing wounds**

Castor oil has special properties that can help wounds heal faster, especially when mixed with other stuff. There's this ointment called Venelex, and it has castor oil and balsam Peru in it. People use it to treat skin and pressure wounds.

The oil can stop infections by keeping wounds moist, and it also has something called ricinoleic acid that helps with swelling.

But, don't use castor oil on small cuts or burns at home. Save it for when a doctor or hospital recommends it for wound care.

- **Skin benefits**

Castor oil is packed with fatty acids, making it great for keeping your skin moisturized. You'll see it listed in the ingredients of various beauty products you buy. You can even use it by itself in its natural state, without any added scents or colors. Just be careful, as it might irritate your skin, so it's a good idea to mix it with another gentle oil.

Some folks believe that castor oil's antibacterial, anti-inflammatory, and moisturizing properties could be useful against acne. However, there isn't any research to support this idea.

- **Hair growth**

Castor oil is often promoted as a remedy for dry scalp, hair growth, and dandruff. Some people believe it can moisturize the scalp and hair. However, there is no scientific evidence supporting the idea that it effectively treats dandruff or encourages hair growth.

In reality, using castor oil on your hair might lead to a rare problem called felting. This occurs when your hair gets so tangled that it has to be cut off.

Historical significance

As people often say, history tends to repeat itself. This happens, especially when we don't pay attention to the lessons passed down by our elders, the wise individuals who came before us. These experienced individuals have shared valuable insights that are like hidden treasures, easily accessible if we take a closer look. These treasures offer practical guidance on living well and help us avoid making mistakes in our lives.

Castor oil is like a hidden gem for our health.

If you've been exploring natural health remedies, you've probably come across this well-known oil. Maybe you've spotted it on the bottom shelf of health food stores. This oil has a long history and is celebrated in various cultures. It's proven to be incredibly valuable and can be considered the ultimate healing and beautifying oil. It's a DIY solution that's both natural and affordable, making it a standout choice in the world of health and beauty.

People started using castor oil around 4000 BC, according to findings in Egyptian tombs dug up by archaeologists. That means humans have been using this oil for over 6000 years! The Egyptians used it for embalming dead bodies and also as fuel for lamps. In an ancient medical document called the Ebers Papyrus, they even talked about using castor oil as a laxative.

- **Understanding the Spiritual Significance of Castor Oil**

The name Palma Christi is commonly associated with an oil derived from the castor bean plant. According to belief, this oil was used by Christ in the Bible for anointing the sick. The name "Palma Christi" is given because the leaves of the castor bean plant, from which the oil is ideally cold-pressed, are thought to resemble a healing hand – symbolizing the ultimate healing hand of Christ.

Legend has it that this oil was not only used by Christ but also served as the anointing oil for kings, queens, priests, and priestesses during significant ceremonies. It was believed to have unifying properties with the spirit, potentially fostering a connection with God.

- **History of cosmetic use**

Throughout history, many famous individuals, including Cleopatra, and revered figures like Greek Herodotus and Roman Pliny the Elder, have utilized castor oil for various purposes. Cleopatra used it to enhance the beauty of her eyes, while Greek and Roman Goddesses applied it to improve the health and appearance of their hair, skin, and nails.

In the field of medicine, both Herodotus and Pliny the Elder turned to castor oil for its numerous medicinal benefits. They employed it to address various health issues and noted its effectiveness in skin whitening and promoting hair growth. It's remarkable how such a straightforward oil has found diverse applications over time.

- **A potent anti-inflammatory**

This amazing oil has a unique mix of three key components: Omega 9 oleic acid (found in olive oil), Omega 6 linoleic acid (usually in sesame oil), and a special ingredient called ricinoleic acid. Ricinoleic acid works similarly to the way your body processes fish oil, producing anti-inflammatory prostaglandins. This makes the oil versatile and beneficial for various purposes, like an all-purpose solution for health and beauty, a must-have in your home medicine cabinet.

In the East, Traditional Chinese Medicine documents mention using this oil topically with a compress for swollen joints. This makes sense because of its anti-inflammatory properties. This could be the first-time castor oil was used in this way.

- **Using Castor Oil for Going to the Bathroom, Dealing with Parasites, and... as a Form of Consequence?**

Throughout history, various cultures like those in East India and practitioners of Ayurvedic Medicine have utilized castor oil as a remedy for constipation and digestive issues.

In the Caribbean, as well as in both East and West Indian cultures, castor oil was commonly used as a weekly purgative. People believed it helped cleanse the intestines, prevent parasites, and, in some instances, it was even used as a form of punishment for misbehavior. An interesting example of this can be found in the 1943 MGM cartoon "Baby Puss" from the Tom and Jerry series, where Tom, the cat, feigns being a baby and is given castor oil by Jerry as a consequence for his bad behavior.

Castor oil has also found its place in various ethnobotanical practices worldwide. In some cultures, it has been administered to babies to assist in their first bowel movements.

The dark ages

Like anything good, castor oil has its drawbacks too. In the past, people didn't always use it wisely. In the 19th century in Mexico, there was a time called the 'Empacho' when people would use castor oil excessively after eating and drinking too much, thinking it would cleanse their bodies.

In the 20th century, in Italy during the fascist regime, castor oil took on a darker role. Italian soldiers used it as a form of torture to make people have diarrhea. In some cases, this caused prisoners to lose essential nutrients, leading to serious health issues and even death.

Upgrading Castor Oil for Today's Needs

In the early 1900s in North America, stores that sold medicine and remedies, like apothecaries and pharmacies, had castor oil alongside other natural remedies such as ipecac, senna, and witch hazel.

There was a well-known healer in North America named Edgar Cayce who became famous for promoting the use of castor oil packs. He was a bedside healer who read the King James version of the Bible daily and was known for coming up with treatments for his clients. No matter the health issue, he always included the use of castor oil packs in his treatment plans.

As time passed, this practice gained popularity and became part of the methods used by naturopathic doctors and functional medicine practitioners around the world.

Even in conventional medicine, castor oil is used by midwives and doulas to help induce labor.

The Comeback of Castor Oil for Beautiful Skin and Hair

Lately, there's a growing trend that started in the Mediterranean and Caribbean regions and is now making a comeback. People are using a particular oil for cosmetic purposes, applying it to their hair, eyebrows, and eyelashes to promote growth. This practice has become popular in various parts of the world.

Furthermore, this oil has become the top choice as a carrier for essential oils, which are widely popular globally. The uniqueness of this oil lies in its ability to penetrate the second layer of the skin (dermis), allowing essential oils and other beneficial skin oils to reach deeper into the body.

Why one more book on castor oil?

In the enchanting pages of "The Miracle Elixir: Unlocking the Secrets and Benefits of Castor Oil," embark on a transformative journey into the heart of nature's hidden treasure. Castor oil, a time-honored elixir with a rich history, unfolds its secrets in this comprehensive guide, revealing its remarkable potential to revitalize your health and beauty.

Dive deep into the origins of castor oil, tracing its roots through ancient civilizations and medicinal practices. Explore the science behind its composition and discover how this seemingly simple oil holds the key to a myriad of health and wellness wonders.

This book serves as your trusted companion, offering a treasure trove of insights into the diverse applications of castor oil. From promoting lush, radiant hair and nurturing supple skin to addressing common ailments and supporting overall well-being, the miraculous properties of castor oil are unveiled chapter by chapter.

Immerse yourself in practical tips, easy-to-follow recipes, and real-life success stories that illuminate the transformative power of castor oil. Whether you seek to enhance your beauty routine, boost your immune system, or alleviate discomfort, this guide provides a holistic approach to incorporating castor oil into your daily life.

"The Miracle Elixir" is not just a book; it's a roadmap to harnessing the untapped potential of nature's gift. Join us on a captivating exploration of castor oil's secrets and witness the incredible results that await those who embrace its wonders. Your journey to radiant health and timeless beauty begins here.

Composition & Nutritional Value

Nutritional Value

You can eat castor oil, and in one tablespoon, you get:

- Calories: 120
- Fat: 14 grams

Castor oil also has vitamin E and something called ricinoleic acid, which is a type of healthy fat.

Health Benefits

Castor oil can be beneficial for your health in various ways, both when taken internally and applied externally. Here's a simple breakdown of the advantages:

1. Eases Constipation:

Castor oil acts like a natural laxative, helping to relieve temporary constipation. It works by causing the muscles in the intestines to contract and clear the bowels. A study [1] on older adults found that using castor oil packs reduced constipation symptoms, making bowel movements easier.

2. Reduces Inflammation:

Thanks to ricinoleic acid, castor oil has anti-inflammatory and pain-relieving properties. Applying a gel with ricinoleic acid onto the skin has been shown [2] to reduce pain and inflammation in comparison to other treatments.

3. Moisturizes Skin:

Castor oil, found in cosmetic products like moisturizers, contains hydrating properties. Ricinoleic acid in the oil acts as a humectant, preventing water loss and keeping the skin moisturized. It can be a natural alternative to commercial moisturizers and may benefit those with dry or irritated skin, including those with psoriasis.

4. Promotes Dental Health:

Castor oil's antifungal properties may contribute to improved dental health. It could help combat fungi causing issues like root canal infections and plaque overgrowth. Research suggests it can eliminate the Candida albicans fungus from contaminated root canals [3].

5. Combats Acne:

Castor oil is effective against acne symptoms due to its anti-inflammatory and antimicrobial properties. It can reduce inflammation-related acne symptoms and prevent bacterial growth. Studies indicate that castor oil has been successful in treating acne.

6. Aids in Wound Healing:

Castor oil can help reduce infection risks and promote wound healing. It stimulates tissue growth, reduces dryness, and removes dead skin cells. A study [4] on nursing home residents with ulcers found that an ointment containing castor oil had better healing rates and shorter healing times.

7. Improves Hair Health:

Castor oil is beneficial for dry and damaged hair. Studies [5] show that it moisturizes the hair shaft, decreasing the likelihood of breakage. It also helps moisturize the scalp, reducing dandruff caused by conditions like seborrheic dermatitis.

Health Benefits

Skin care

Castor oil is a versatile and natural remedy that has been used for centuries for various purposes, including skincare. Here are some potential benefits of castor oil for the skin:

- **Moisturizing Properties:**

Castor oil is rich in fatty acids, particularly ricinoleic acid, which has moisturizing properties. It helps to lock in moisture and prevent the skin from becoming dry and flaky.

- **Anti-Inflammatory Effects:**

The anti-inflammatory properties of castor oil can help reduce redness and inflammation on the skin. This makes it potentially beneficial for conditions such as acne, dermatitis, and other inflammatory skin issues.

- **Acne Treatment:**

Castor oil has antimicrobial properties that may help fight bacteria on the skin, making it a potential treatment for acne. It can also help regulate oil production, preventing clogged pores.

- **Scar Reduction:**

Applying castor oil regularly to scars may help reduce their appearance. The oil penetrates deep into the skin layers, promoting the growth of healthy tissue and reducing the visibility of scars over time.

- **Anti-Aging Benefits:**

Castor oil contains antioxidants that can help fight free radicals and prevent premature aging. It may help reduce the appearance of fine lines and wrinkles, promoting a more youthful complexion.

- **Promoting Wound Healing:**

The anti-inflammatory and antibacterial properties of castor oil make it potentially beneficial for promoting the healing of wounds, cuts, and abrasions. It can help prevent infections and soothe irritated skin.

- **Natural Cleanser:**

Castor oil can be used as a natural cleanser to remove impurities and makeup from the skin. It can help dissolve excess oil without stripping the skin of its natural moisture.

- **Eyelash and Eyebrow Growth:**

Some people use castor oil to promote the growth of eyelashes and eyebrows. Applying a small amount to these areas may help nourish the hair follicles and encourage thicker, longer hair growth.

- **Preventing Stretch Marks:**

Pregnant women often use castor oil to prevent and minimize stretch marks. Its moisturizing properties can help keep the skin supple and elastic.

- **Soothing Sunburns:**

The anti-inflammatory properties of castor oil may help soothe sunburned skin. Applying a thin layer can provide relief and aid in the healing process.

How to Use

- For general skincare, apply a small amount of castor oil to clean, dry skin and massage gently.

- For acne-prone skin, mix castor oil with a carrier oil like jojoba or coconut oil to avoid clogging pores.

- Use a patch test before applying it to a larger area to ensure you don't have an allergic reaction.

- It's advisable to choose cold-pressed and organic castor oil for skincare to ensure purity.

While castor oil has various potential benefits for the skin, individual reactions may vary. If you have sensitive skin or are unsure about using castor oil, it's advisable to consult with a dermatologist before incorporating it into your skincare routine.

Hair care

- **Promotes Hair Growth:**

Castor oil is rich in ricinoleic acid, which has anti-inflammatory and antimicrobial properties. These properties can help to keep the scalp healthy, potentially improving hair growth.

- **Strengthens Hair:**

The nutrients in castor oil, such as vitamin E, minerals, and proteins, can help strengthen the hair shaft, preventing breakage and split ends.

- **Prevents Hair Loss:**

By nourishing the hair follicles and strengthening the roots, castor oil may help prevent hair loss. It works by improving blood circulation to the scalp and providing essential nutrients to the hair follicles.

- **Conditions and Moisturizes:**

Castor oil is a thick and rich oil, making it an excellent natural conditioner. It helps moisturize the hair, making it softer and more manageable.

- **Treats Scalp Infections:**

The antimicrobial properties of castor oil can help in treating scalp infections and dandruff, promoting a healthier scalp environment for hair growth.

- **Prevents Premature Graying:**

Regular application of castor oil may help slow down the process of premature graying by providing essential nutrients to the hair follicles and promoting overall hair health.

- **Adds Shine to Hair:**

Castor oil can add a natural shine to the hair, making it look healthier and more vibrant.

- **Reduces Split Ends:**

The conditioning properties of castor oil help in reducing split ends by moisturizing and nourishing the hair shaft.

- **Thickens Hair:**

Regular use of castor oil can contribute to thicker hair, as it helps in strengthening the hair shaft and promoting overall hair health.

- **Improves Blood Circulation:**

Massaging castor oil into the scalp can improve blood circulation, which is beneficial for hair growth as it ensures that hair follicles receive an adequate supply of nutrients.

- **Natural Humectant:**

Castor oil is a natural humectant, which means it helps to lock in moisture. This can be especially beneficial for individuals with dry or damaged hair.

- **Split End Treatment:**

Applying castor oil to the ends of the hair can help in repairing split ends, giving the hair a smoother and healthier appearance.

To use castor oil for hair, you can apply it directly to your scalp and hair, massage it in, and leave it on for at least 30 minutes before washing it out. Some people prefer to mix it with other oils or incorporate it into homemade hair masks for enhanced benefits. Always perform a patch test before using any new product, especially if you have sensitive skin or allergies.

Joint and muscle pain relief

While scientific research on its effectiveness for joint and muscle pain relief is somewhat limited, some anecdotal evidence and traditional uses suggest potential benefits. Here are some of the ways in which castor oil may be beneficial for joint and muscle pain:

- **Anti-inflammatory Properties:**

Castor oil contains ricinoleic acid, which is known for its anti-inflammatory properties. Inflammation is a common cause of joint and muscle pain, and reducing inflammation can help alleviate discomfort.

- **Analgesic (Pain-Relieving) Effects:**

The anti-inflammatory properties of castor oil may contribute to its analgesic effects. By reducing inflammation, castor oil may help to relieve pain associated with joint and muscle conditions.

- **Improved Blood Circulation:**

Massaging castor oil onto the affected joints or muscles can promote better blood circulation. Improved blood flow can facilitate the delivery of oxygen and nutrients to the affected area, promoting healing and reducing pain.

- **Joint Lubrication:**

Applying castor oil topically may provide a lubricating effect on the joints, potentially easing stiffness and enhancing flexibility. This can be particularly beneficial for individuals with arthritis or other joint-related conditions.

- **Detoxification:**

Castor oil packs, which involve applying a cloth soaked in castor oil to the affected area, are a popular traditional remedy. Some believe that these packs can help detoxify the body by stimulating lymphatic circulation, which may indirectly contribute to pain relief.

- **Muscle Relaxation:**

Massaging castor oil onto sore muscles may help relax them, providing relief from muscle tension and spasms. This can be especially beneficial for individuals experiencing muscle pain due to overuse or strain.

- **Moisturizing and Nourishing:**

Castor oil has moisturizing properties that can help nourish the skin and underlying tissues. Proper hydration of the skin and tissues can contribute to overall joint and muscle health.

- **Cost-Effective and Accessible:**

Castor oil is relatively affordable and widely available, making it a convenient option for individuals seeking natural remedies for joint and muscle pain.

It's important to note that while many people find relief using castor oil, individual responses may vary.

If you have persistent or severe joint and muscle pain, it's advisable to consult with a healthcare professional for a proper diagnosis and guidance on the most appropriate treatment for your specific condition. Additionally, if you have allergies or skin sensitivities, it's recommended to perform a patch test before applying castor oil topically to ensure you don't have any adverse reactions.

Gastrointestinal health

While castor oil is often associated with its use as a laxative, its impact on gastrointestinal health goes beyond just promoting bowel movements. It's essential to note that while castor oil may have some potential benefits for gastrointestinal health, its use should be approached with caution, and it's always advisable to consult with a healthcare professional before using it as a remedy. Here are some potential benefits of castor oil on gastrointestinal health:

- **Laxative Effect:**

Castor oil is a well-known natural laxative. It works by increasing the movement of the muscles in the intestines, which helps facilitate the passing of stool.

The active component responsible for this effect is ricinoleic acid, which stimulates the smooth muscle cells in the intestines, promoting bowel movements.

- **Constipation Relief:**

Due to its laxative properties, castor oil can be effective in providing relief from occasional constipation.

It is often used as a short-term remedy for constipation, but it should not be used regularly or in excess, as it can lead to dehydration and electrolyte imbalance.

- **Anti-Inflammatory Properties:**

Ricinoleic acid, the main fatty acid in castor oil, exhibits anti-inflammatory effects. Inflammation in the gastrointestinal tract can contribute to various digestive issues.

By reducing inflammation, castor oil may help alleviate symptoms associated with conditions like irritable bowel syndrome (IBS) or inflammatory bowel diseases (IBD).

- **Promotion of Detoxification:**

Some proponents suggest that castor oil may aid in detoxification by promoting the elimination of waste from the body.

It is believed to stimulate the liver, enhancing its ability to filter toxins and promoting the elimination of waste through the digestive system.

- **Microbial Balance:**

Castor oil has demonstrated antimicrobial properties in some studies, which may help in maintaining a healthy balance of microorganisms in the gut.

Maintaining a balanced gut microbiota is crucial for digestive health and overall well-being.

- **Potential Anti-Cancer Effects:**

Some preclinical studies have explored the potential anti-cancer properties of components found in castor oil, suggesting that it may have a role in preventing or slowing the growth of certain cancer cells.

However, more research is needed in this area, and it is not advisable to rely on castor oil as a primary cancer prevention strategy.

It's important to note that while castor oil may offer certain benefits, its use as a remedy should be done cautiously. Excessive or prolonged use of castor oil as a laxative can lead to dehydration, electrolyte imbalance, and dependence on laxatives. Additionally, individual responses to castor oil can vary, and some people may experience adverse effects. Always consult with a healthcare professional before using castor oil or any other natural remedy for gastrointestinal issues.

Medical Applications

The Laxative Function

One of the most well-known uses of castor oil for health is its natural ability to help with constipation.

Think of castor oil as a quick-acting solution for occasional constipation. It falls under the category of stimulative laxatives, meaning it speeds up the muscles in your intestines to move things along and clear your bowels. The Food and Drug Administration (FDA) approves castor oil for use as a stimulative laxative.

Here's a simple explanation of how it works: When you swallow castor oil, it gets broken down in your small intestine, releasing a fatty acid called ricinoleic acid. This acid is absorbed by your intestines and triggers a strong laxative effect.

Studies have shown that castor oil can effectively relieve constipation. For instance, a study in 2011 found that older adults who took castor oil experienced reduced symptoms of constipation, like less straining during bowel movements and fewer feelings of incomplete bowel movements.

Another study demonstrated that castor oil was successful in clearing people's bowels before a noninvasive colonoscopy called a colon capsule endoscopy.

While castor oil is generally safe in small amounts, taking too much can lead to stomach cramps, nausea, vomiting, and diarrhea.

It's important to note that although castor oil can help with occasional constipation, it's not recommended for long-term use. Before using castor oil to treat constipation, consult with a healthcare professional. Misusing castor oil can have serious side effects, including life-threatening issues like electrolyte and acid-base imbalances.

A Natural Moisturizer

Castor oil is a natural substance that contains a special type of fat called ricinoleic acid, which is good for your skin. This fat helps keep your skin moisturized by forming a protective barrier that prevents water from escaping.

Cosmetic companies use castor oil in products like lotions and makeup to make your skin more hydrated. You can also use castor oil by itself instead of store-bought moisturizers. Many of those products have potentially harmful ingredients like preservatives and perfumes that can irritate your skin.

By using castor oil, you can avoid these additives, and it's also affordable. You can apply it to both your face and body.

Castor oil is thick, so some people mix it with other oils like almond, olive, or coconut oil to create a super-hydrating moisturizer. While castor oil is generally safe for most people, it might cause an allergic reaction in some. To be safe, you can mix it with another oil like jojoba or coconut oil and test a small amount on a small area of skin before using it on larger areas.

Castor Oil May Make Your Wounds to Heal Faster

Putting castor oil on wounds keeps them moist, which can help them heal and prevent them from drying out.

Venelex, a popular ointment used in hospitals to treat wounds, has both castor oil and Peru balsam (made from the Myroxylon balsamum tree). It's used for chronic and acute wounds, like pressure ulcers, diabetic ulcers, burns, and surgical wounds. Venelex reduces odors, protects wounds, and creates a moist environment to aid healing.

The main fatty acid in castor oil, ricinoleic acid, has anti-inflammatory and pain-reducing properties. It can help with skin inflammation, support healing, and reduce pain for people with wounds.

Studies show that ointments with castor oil can effectively treat various wounds. In a 2013 case study, a spray with Peru balsam, castor oil, and an enzyme called trypsin helped heal a surgical wound in an 81-

year-old man who couldn't tolerate other topical therapies.

Remember, castor oil wound treatments have multiple ingredients, not just castor oil. Always consult a healthcare professional before applying castor oil to any wound.

Could be useful for keeping dentures clean and safe when not in use

Bacteria and fungi, like Candida, often grow on dentures. If dentures aren't cleaned properly, it can cause oral problems.

Candida, a type of fungus, is a big issue for denture wearers because it easily sticks to dentures and the mouth.

Too much Candida can cause a condition called denture stomatitis, which leads to inflammation and irritation in the mouth.

Interestingly, using castor oil to clean dentures might help prevent denture stomatitis because castor oil can kill bacteria and fungi.

A study found that soaking dentures in a solution with 10% castor oil for 20 minutes reduced Candida and other harmful bacteria.

In 2013, a study on older people with denture-related stomatitis found that using a castor oil mouthwash improved the signs of stomatitis, including inflammation.

Another study showed that brushing and soaking dentures in a castor oil solution significantly reduced Candida in older denture wearers.

Unveiling the Elegance of Castor Oil in Beauty and Personal Care

In the pursuit of natural beauty and self-care, castor oil emerges as a versatile elixir, offering a multitude of benefits for the skin, hair, and overall well-being. This chapter delves into the diverse applications of castor oil in beauty and personal care, exploring natural skincare recipes, castor oil cleaning routines, DIY facemasks, homemade hair treatments, deep conditioning, and scalp massage techniques.

Natural skincare recipes

- **Castor oil cleansing balm**

Castor oil cleansing balm is a skincare product designed to cleanse the skin by removing makeup, dirt, and impurities. Castor oil, known for its moisturizing and cleansing properties, is a key ingredient in this type of balm. The balm is formulated to be gentle on the skin while effectively breaking down and removing makeup and other debris.

Here are some key points about castor oil cleansing balm:

Ingredients

Castor Oil: Castor oil is the star ingredient, known for its ability to deeply cleanse the skin without stripping it of natural oils. It also has moisturizing properties.

Other Oils: Many formulations include additional oils such as olive oil, jojoba oil, or almond oil. These oils help to nourish and hydrate the skin.

Cleansing Process

Oil-Based Cleansing: Castor oil cleansing balms work on the principle that like dissolves like. The oils in the balm help to dissolve and lift away the oils in makeup and impurities on the skin.

Gentle Emulsification: When the balm comes into contact with water during rinsing, it emulsifies, turning into a milky texture. This makes it easy to rinse away, leaving the skin feeling clean.

Benefits

Effective Makeup Removal: Castor oil cleansing balms are particularly effective in breaking down and removing waterproof makeup and sunscreen.

Moisturizing: The balm helps maintain the skin's natural moisture balance, preventing over-drying.

Gentle Exfoliation: Some formulations may contain ingredients that offer mild exfoliation, promoting a smoother complexion.

Skin Types

All Skin Types: Castor oil cleansing balms are generally suitable for all skin types, including sensitive and dry skin.

Balancing: The cleansing balm can help balance the skin by removing excess oils without causing dryness.

How to Use

Application: Take a small amount of the balm and massage it onto dry skin with gentle, circular motions.

Emulsification: Add a little water to emulsify the balm, turning it into a milky texture.

Rinsing: Rinse thoroughly with water or use a damp cloth to wipe away the emulsified balm.

Caution

Patch Test: It's advisable to perform a patch test before using any new skincare product to ensure compatibility with your skin.

Avoid Eye Area: While effective for removing makeup, be cautious around the eye area to prevent irritation.

Castor oil cleansing balms offer a luxurious and effective way to cleanse the skin, leaving it feeling soft, hydrated, and refreshed. As with any skincare product, individual reactions may vary, so it's essential to choose products that suit your specific skin needs.

- **Moisturizing castor oil serum**

Ingredients

Castor Oil:

2 tablespoons of organic, cold-pressed castor oil.

Carrier Oil (Optional):

1 tablespoon of a lighter carrier oil like jojoba oil, coconut oil, or sweet almond oil. This helps dilute the thick consistency of castor oil and makes it easier to apply.

Essential Oils (Optional):

5-10 drops of essential oils such as lavender, rosemary, or peppermint for added fragrance and potential benefits for hair and scalp.

Instructions

Select Your Ingredients:

Choose high-quality, organic castor oil for the best results. If you decide to use a carrier oil, pick one that complements your hair and skin type.

Measure and Mix:

In a small bowl or a clean container, measure 2 tablespoons of castor oil. If you're using a carrier oil, add 1 tablespoon as well. Mix the oils thoroughly.

Add Essential Oils (Optional):

If you want to enhance the scent and potential benefits of your serum, add 5-10 drops of your chosen essential oil. Stir well to ensure even distribution.

Transfer to an Applicator Bottle:

Use a small funnel to transfer the mixture into a dark glass applicator bottle. Dark glass helps protect the oil from sunlight, preserving its properties.

Application

Apply the Castor Oil Serum to your hair or skin as needed. For hair, focus on the roots and tips. For the skin, gently massage a small amount onto the desired area.

Leave-In or Wash Out:

You can leave the serum in overnight for an intensive treatment, or if used during the day, leave it on for at least 30 minutes before washing it out.

Frequency:

Use the Castor Oil Serum 1-2 times a week for best results. Adjust the frequency based on your individual needs and preferences.

Storage

Store the serum in a cool, dark place. Shake well before each use, as natural oils may separate over time.

Remember to do a patch test before applying the serum to a larger area to ensure you don't have any adverse reactions. Enjoy the nourishing benefits of this DIY Castor Oil Serum for healthier-looking hair and skin!

- **Castor oil and honey exfoliator**

Castor oil and honey can be combined to create a natural and effective exfoliator that promotes smooth and healthy skin. Both ingredients offer unique benefits that contribute to the overall well-being of your skin.

Properties of Honey

Natural Humectant: Honey is a natural humectant, meaning it attracts and retains moisture. This makes it an excellent ingredient for hydrating the skin.

Antioxidant Properties: Honey contains antioxidants that help protect the skin from damage caused by free radicals. This can contribute to a youthful and radiant complexion.

Antibacterial and Antimicrobial: Honey has natural antibacterial and antimicrobial properties, making it effective in preventing and treating acne.

Gentle Exfoliation: The enzymes present in honey help to gently exfoliate the skin, removing dead skin cells and promoting a smoother texture.

Castor Oil and Honey Exfoliator Recipe:

Ingredients:

1 tablespoon castor oil

1 tablespoon raw honey

Instructions:

Mixing: In a small bowl, combine the castor oil and raw honey. Stir well to ensure the ingredients are thoroughly blended.

Application: Apply the mixture to your face in a gentle, circular motion. Avoid the eye area.

Massage: Gently massage the exfoliator into your skin for about 2-3 minutes. The granules in honey provide a mild exfoliation, helping to remove dead skin cells.

Rinse: Rinse your face with warm water to remove the exfoliator. Pat your skin dry with a clean towel.

Moisturize: Follow up with your regular moisturizer to lock in the hydration.

***Note:** Perform a patch test before applying any new mixture to your face to ensure you do not have an adverse reaction.

This natural exfoliator can be used once or twice a week, depending on your skin type. Regular use can leave your skin feeling soft, moisturized, and rejuvenated.

Castor oil cleansing routine

Incorporating castor oil into your cleaning routine can help cleanse and nourish your skin. Here's a step-by-step guide on how to use castor oil in your cleaning routine:

Choose Cold-Pressed, Hexane-Free Castor Oil:

Select a high-quality, cold-pressed castor oil that is free from hexane, ensuring that you get the purest form of the oil for your skincare routine.

Gather Your Supplies:

- Castor oil
- Carrier oil (optional, such as olive oil or almond oil)
- Soft washcloth
- Warm water

Perform a Patch Test:

Before incorporating castor oil into your routine, perform a patch test on a small area of your skin to ensure you don't have any adverse reactions.

Create a Castor Oil Blend (Optional):

If castor oil feels too thick on its own, you can create a blend by mixing it with a lighter carrier oil, like olive oil or almond oil. This helps make the application smoother.

Start with a Dry Face:

Begin with a dry face, free from makeup and impurities. Tie back your hair to keep it away from your face during the cleansing process.

Apply Castor Oil to Your Face:

Take a small amount of castor oil or your castor oil blend onto your fingertips.

Gently massage the oil onto your face using circular motions. Focus on areas with makeup or impurities.

Massage and Cleanse:

Spend a few minutes massaging the oil into your skin. This helps dissolve makeup, dirt, and excess oil.

The massaging action also promotes blood circulation, contributing to a healthy complexion.

Use a Warm Washcloth:

Soak a soft washcloth in warm water.

Wring out excess water and place the warm washcloth over your face. Allow it to sit for a moment to open up your pores.

Gently Wipe Away the Oil:

Use the washcloth to gently wipe away the oil from your face. The warm cloth helps to remove impurities effectively.

Repeat if Necessary:

If you wear heavy makeup or sunscreen, you may need to repeat the process to ensure thorough cleansing.

Follow with Your Regular Skincare Routine:

After cleansing with castor oil, follow up with your usual toner, serum, and moisturizer to lock in hydration.

Frequency:

You can incorporate this routine into your skincare regimen a few times a week or as needed, depending on your skin type.

Adjust Based on Your Skin's Response:

Monitor how your skin responds to the castor oil cleaning routine. Adjust the frequency and the amount of oil used based on your skin's needs.

Remember that everyone's skin is different, and it may take some time to find the right balance for your individual needs. If you experience any irritation or discomfort, discontinue use and consult with a dermatologist.

DIY Facemasks

- **Detoxifying Clay Mask with Castor Oil**

A detoxifying clay mask with castor oil can be a beneficial addition to your skincare routine, offering a natural and effective way to cleanse and rejuvenate your skin. Clay masks are renowned for their ability to draw out impurities, excess oils, and toxins from the skin, while castor oil provides nourishment and promotes a healthy complexion. Here's a simple recipe and a guide on how to create and use a detoxifying clay mask with castor oil:

Ingredients

1. Bentonite clay - 2 tablespoons

2. Activated charcoal powder - 1 teaspoon

3. Apple cider vinegar - 1 tablespoon (or enough to make a paste)

4. Castor oil - 1 teaspoon

5. Optional: Essential oils (such as tea tree oil or lavender oil) - a few drops

Instructions

Prepare the Mixture:

In a non-metallic bowl, combine the bentonite clay and activated charcoal powder.

Add Liquids:

Slowly add apple cider vinegar to the dry ingredients while stirring to create a smooth paste. Adjust the amount of vinegar to achieve the desired consistency.

Incorporate Castor Oil:

Add castor oil to the mixture and blend well. Castor oil helps balance the drying effects of clay, providing hydration to the skin.

Optional: Essential Oils:

If desired, add a few drops of essential oils like tea tree or lavender. These oils can add fragrance and provide additional skin benefits.

Mix Thoroughly:

Stir the mixture until all ingredients are well combined. Ensure that there are no lumps in the paste.

How to Use

Cleanse Your Face:

Start with a clean face. Gently wash your face to remove any makeup, dirt, or excess oils.

Apply the Mask:

Using a clean brush or your fingertips, apply an even layer of the clay mask to your face, avoiding the delicate eye area.

Relax and Let it Dry:

Allow the mask to dry for about 10-15 minutes. As it dries, you may feel a tightening sensation.

Rinse Off:

Once the mask is fully dry, rinse it off with lukewarm water. Use gentle circular motions to exfoliate as you remove the mask.

Moisturize:

Pat your face dry and follow up with a lightweight, hydrating moisturizer to lock in moisture.

Benefits

Detoxification: Bentonite clay and activated charcoal help absorb toxins and impurities from the skin.

Nourishment: Castor oil provides essential fatty acids and antioxidants, promoting skin health.

Balancing: The combination of ingredients helps balance excess oil production without overly drying the skin.

Skin Rejuvenation: Regular use can contribute to a clearer complexion, reduced breakouts, and a revitalized skin appearance.

- **Soothing Aloe Vera and Castor Oil Mask**

In the realm of natural skincare, Aloe Vera and Castor Oil stand out as formidable allies for achieving radiant and healthy skin. When combined in a harmonious blend, these two botanical powerhouses create a soothing and nourishing mask that can work wonders for your complexion. Let's delve into the benefits of this rejuvenating concoction and learn how to make a simple yet effective Aloe Vera and Castor Oil mask for a spa-like treat at home.

Benefits of Aloe Vera and Castor Oil for the Skin

Aloe Vera

Hydration: Aloe Vera is renowned for its exceptional moisturizing properties. It deeply hydrates the skin, leaving it supple and revitalized.

Soothing: The gel from Aloe Vera is known for its anti-inflammatory and cooling effects, making it ideal for calming irritated or sunburned skin.

Antioxidant-rich: Aloe Vera contains antioxidants that help combat free radicals, preventing premature aging and promoting a youthful complexion.

Castor Oil

Deep Nourishment: Castor oil is rich in fatty acids that nourish the skin, providing a natural boost to its texture and elasticity.

Anti-Inflammatory: Its anti-inflammatory properties can reduce redness and swelling, making it suitable for those with sensitive or inflamed skin.

Detoxification: Castor oil aids in the removal of impurities from the skin, promoting a clearer complexion.

DIY Aloe Vera and Castor Oil Mask Recipe

Ingredients:

2 tablespoons of Aloe Vera gel (freshly extracted or store-bought)

1 tablespoon of Castor Oil

Instructions:

1. In a clean bowl, combine the Aloe Vera gel and Castor Oil.

2. Mix the ingredients thoroughly until you achieve a smooth and consistent blend.

3. Cleanse your face to remove any makeup or impurities.

4. Using clean fingertips or a brush, apply the mask evenly to your face, avoiding the eye area.

5. Allow the mask to sit for 15-20 minutes, allowing the potent combination of Aloe Vera and Castor Oil to work its magic.

6. Rinse the mask off with lukewarm water and pat your face dry.

Tips:

Perform a patch test before applying the mask to ensure you don't have any adverse reactions.

Use this mask 1-2 times a week for best results.

Follow up with your regular moisturizer to lock in the hydration.

Indulging in a soothing Aloe Vera and Castor Oil mask offers a luxurious and natural way to pamper your skin. With their combined benefits, this DIY mask can become a staple in your skincare routine, providing hydration, soothing relief, and a radiant glow. Incorporate this simple yet effective treatment into your self-care regimen and let the healing powers of nature enhance the beauty of your skin.

- **Brightening Turmeric and Castor Oil Masks**

A brightening turmeric and castor oil mask is a popular natural skincare remedy that combines the potent properties of turmeric and castor oil to promote healthy and radiant skin. Both ingredients are known for their numerous skincare benefits, making this mask a favorite for those seeking a natural and effective way to enhance their complexion.

Ingredients

Turmeric Powder:

Turmeric is renowned for its anti-inflammatory and antioxidant properties. It helps reduce inflammation, soothe irritated skin, and fight free radicals, contributing to a brighter and more even skin tone.

Castor Oil:

Castor oil is rich in fatty acids and has moisturizing properties. It nourishes the skin, improves its texture, and helps fade dark spots. The oil also possesses antimicrobial properties, making it beneficial for acne-prone skin.

Yogurt or Honey (optional):

Yogurt contains lactic acid, which gently exfoliates the skin and promotes cell turnover. Honey is known for its antibacterial and moisturizing properties. Both ingredients can enhance the mask's overall effectiveness.

Instructions:

In a bowl, combine:

- 1 teaspoon of turmeric powder
- 1 tablespoon of castor oil
- Optionally, add 1 tablespoon of yogurt or honey for additional benefits.

Mix well until you achieve a smooth paste. Adjust the consistency by adding more turmeric or oil if needed.

Cleanse your face thoroughly to remove any makeup, dirt, or impurities.

Apply an even layer of the turmeric and castor oil mask to your face, avoiding the delicate eye area.

Allow the mask to sit for about 15-20 minutes. During this time, you may feel a slight warming sensation due to the turmeric.

Gently rinse off the mask using warm water. Use a soft cloth or your hands to avoid staining.

Follow up with your regular skincare routine, such as applying a moisturizer or serum.

Benefits

Brightening: Turmeric helps lighten dark spots and hyperpigmentation, giving the skin a brighter and more radiant appearance.

Anti-Inflammatory: Turmeric's anti-inflammatory properties can soothe irritated skin and reduce redness.

Moisturizing: Castor oil is deeply moisturizing, making the mask suitable for dry skin types.

Antibacterial: The combination of turmeric and castor oil provides antimicrobial benefits, beneficial for those with acne-prone skin.

Exfoliation (optional): If yogurt is included, the lactic acid helps gently exfoliate the skin, promoting a smoother complexion.

Note

Perform a patch test before applying the mask to ensure you don't have any adverse reactions.

Turmeric may stain clothing, so wear an old shirt or use a dark-colored towel during application.

Consult with a dermatologist if you have specific skin concerns or conditions.

Deep Conditioning

Deep conditioning with castor oil is a popular and effective method to promote hair health and hydration. Castor oil is derived from the seeds of the castor plant (Ricinus communis) and is known for its rich composition of fatty acids, minerals, and vitamins. When used for deep conditioning, castor oil can help nourish the hair, strengthen the strands, and improve overall hair texture. Here's a guide on how to deep condition your hair using castor oil:

Materials Needed

Castor Oil:

Choose cold-pressed, hexane-free castor oil for the best results. This type of castor oil retains more nutrients and is considered more beneficial for hair.

Carrier Oil (Optional):

You can mix castor oil with a lighter carrier oil like coconut oil, olive oil, or almond oil to enhance its spreadability and make it easier to apply.

Shower Cap or Plastic Wrap:

This helps to create a warm environment, allowing the oil to penetrate the hair shaft more effectively.

Towel:

To protect your clothing and surroundings.

Steps for Deep Conditioning with Castor Oil

Prepare the Mixture:

If you're using a carrier oil, mix it with castor oil in a bowl. Adjust the ratio based on your hair's needs.

Section Your Hair:

Divide your hair into manageable sections. This ensures even distribution of the oil and thorough coverage.

Apply the Oil:

Dip your fingers in the oil mixture and apply it to your scalp, massaging gently with circular motions. Ensure that the oil is evenly distributed from roots to tips.

Focus on the Ends:

Pay extra attention to the ends of your hair, which tend to be drier and more prone to damage. Apply more oil to these areas.

Comb Through:

Use a wide-tooth comb to distribute the oil further and detangle your hair. This also helps in ensuring that the oil reaches every strand.

Wrap Your Hair:

Cover your hair with a shower cap or plastic wrap. This creates a warm environment, allowing the oil to penetrate the hair shaft. You can also use a warm towel for added heat.

Leave it in:

Leave the oil in your hair for at least 30 minutes to an hour. For a more intense treatment, you can leave it overnight.

Shampoo and Condition:

Wash your hair with a mild sulfate-free shampoo to remove the oil. Follow up with a moisturizing conditioner.

Repeat:

Depending on your hair's condition, repeat this deep conditioning treatment once a week or as needed.

Benefits of Deep Conditioning with Castor Oil

Moisture Retention:

Castor oil helps seal in moisture, preventing dryness and promoting hydration.

Hair Strength:

The fatty acids in castor oil contribute to hair strength, reducing breakage and split ends.

Improved Scalp Health:

Massaging castor oil into the scalp can enhance circulation, promoting a healthier scalp environment.

Enhanced Shine:

Regular use of castor oil can add a natural shine to your hair.

Stimulates Hair Growth:

Some people believe that castor oil may promote hair growth, though scientific evidence on this is limited.

Deep conditioning with castor oil is a natural and cost-effective way to improve the overall health and appearance of your hair. Consistency is key, so incorporate it into your hair care routine to reap the maximum benefits over time.

Scalp massage techniques

Scalp massage with castor oil is a popular natural remedy believed to promote hair health and stimulate growth. Castor oil is rich in nutrients, including omega-6 fatty acids, vitamin E, and proteins, which can nourish the hair follicles and strengthen the hair shaft. When combined with the therapeutic benefits of a scalp massage, it can create a relaxing and rejuvenating experience for your scalp and hair. Here's a guide on how to perform a scalp massage with castor oil:

Materials Needed

Castor Oil: Choose a high-quality, cold-pressed castor oil for maximum benefits.

Applicator or Dropper: This helps in applying the oil evenly to your scalp.

Wide-Tooth Comb: To detangle your hair before the massage.

Towel or Old T-shirt: To protect your clothing from the oil.

Steps for Scalp Massage with Castor Oil

Prepare the Castor Oil:

Pour a small amount of castor oil into a bowl. Warm the oil slightly by placing the bowl in hot water for a few minutes. This is optional but can enhance the massage experience.

Detangle Your Hair:

Use a wide-tooth comb to gently detangle your hair and remove any knots or tangles.

Section Your Hair:

Divide your hair into manageable sections. This makes it easier to apply the castor oil to the scalp.

Apply Castor Oil to the Scalp:

Use an applicator or dropper to apply the castor oil directly to your scalp. Start at the front and work your way to the back, ensuring even coverage.

Massage Your Scalp:

With the pads of your fingers, start massaging your scalp using circular motions. Apply gentle to moderate pressure, focusing on areas where you want to promote hair growth or have dryness.

Cover Your Hair:

Once your scalp is well-massaged, distribute the remaining oil through the length of your hair. You can use a comb for even distribution.

Wrap Your Hair:

Tie your hair into a loose bun or use a shower cap to cover your hair. This helps to retain heat, allowing the oil to penetrate the hair shaft and nourish the scalp.

Leave it on:

Leave the castor oil on your scalp for at least 30 minutes to an hour. For deeper conditioning, you can leave it overnight.

Wash Your Hair:

Shampoo your hair thoroughly to remove the oil. You might need to shampoo twice to ensure all the oil is washed out.

Repeat:

For optimal results, incorporate this scalp massage with castor oil into your hair care routine once or twice a week.

Regular scalp massages with castor oil can not only improve hair texture and strength but also provide a relaxing self-care ritual. Keep in mind that individual results may vary, and it's essential to be consistent with the routine to see the best results over time.

Risks and Precautions of Castor Oil

Allergic Reactions to Castor Oil

Allergic reactions to castor oil are rare but can occur. Individuals with a known allergy to castor beans or any of its components should exercise caution when using castor oil. Symptoms of an allergic reaction may include:

- Skin rash or hives
- Itching or swelling
- Shortness of breath
- Chest pain
- Dizziness or fainting

If any of these symptoms occur, it is crucial to seek immediate medical attention. In severe cases, an allergic reaction can lead to anaphylaxis, a life-threatening condition that requires emergency intervention.

Dosage Guidelines

Determining the appropriate dosage of castor oil is essential to avoid potential adverse effects. It is important to note that castor oil is primarily used externally for various purposes, such as skin conditions, massage, and promoting hair growth. However, it can also be ingested for its laxative properties.

External Use:

Skin Conditions: Apply a small amount to the affected area and massage gently. Perform a patch test before widespread use to ensure there is no adverse reaction.

Hair Growth: Mix with a carrier oil and apply to the scalp. Leave it on for a specific duration (as indicated in the product instructions) before washing thoroughly.

Internal Use (Laxative):

Adults: Start with 1 to 2 teaspoons and observe the effects. Dosage can be adjusted based on individual response.

Children: Consult a healthcare professional for appropriate dosage based on age and weight.

It is essential to follow the recommended guidelines and consult a healthcare provider, especially when considering internal use for its laxative effects, as misuse can lead to dehydration and electrolyte imbalances.

Safe Application Guidelines

To maximize the benefits of castor oil while minimizing risks, adherence to safe application guidelines is crucial:

Quality Matters: Choose a high-quality, cold-pressed castor oil to ensure it is free from impurities and contaminants.

Patch Test: Before widespread application, conduct a patch test on a small area of skin to check for allergic reactions.

Dilution: If using castor oil for massage or hair growth, consider diluting it with a carrier oil to prevent skin irritation.

Follow Instructions: Adhere to product-specific instructions regarding application duration, frequency, and any other recommendations.

In conclusion, while castor oil offers numerous health benefits, users must be aware of the potential risks and take necessary precautions. It is advisable to consult with a healthcare professional before incorporating castor oil into a regular health or beauty regimen, especially for those with pre-existing medical conditions or allergies. By following recommended guidelines, individuals can harness the therapeutic properties of castor oil safely and effectively.

Choosing the Right Castor Oil

Understanding Types of Castor Oil

Castor oil comes in different types, each with its unique properties. The three primary types are:

Cold-Pressed Castor Oil: Extracted by pressing castor beans without heat, this type retains more nutrients and is often considered superior.

Jamaican Black Castor Oil (JBCO): Known for its dark color and distinctive roasted scent, JBCO undergoes a different extraction process, involving roasting the beans before pressing.

Hydrogenated Castor Oil: This type undergoes hydrogenation to improve stability, but it may lack some of the beneficial properties found in cold-pressed varieties.

Check for Purity

When choosing castor oil, opt for products that are 100% pure and free from additives or fillers. Read the label carefully to ensure there are no additional ingredients that could dilute the oil's effectiveness.

Look for Organic and Hexane-Free:

Organic castor oil is produced without synthetic pesticides, ensuring a purer product. Additionally, choose castor oil that is hexane-free, as this chemical solvent can leave residue in the oil, affecting its quality.

Consider the Extraction Method

The extraction method plays a crucial role in determining the oil's quality. Cold-pressed castor oil is preferred, as it preserves the oil's natural properties and nutrients. Look for products that explicitly mention the extraction method on the label.

Assess Color and Odor

High-quality castor oil is typically pale yellow or colorless with a mild, nutty aroma. Be cautious if the oil has a strong, unpleasant odor or if it is excessively dark, as this may indicate impurities or over-processing.

Packaging Matters

Castor oil is sensitive to light and air, which can cause it to degrade over time. Choose products that come in dark glass bottles or opaque containers to protect the oil from light. Additionally, opt for bottles with a secure cap to prevent air exposure.

Consider Your Purpose

Different grades of castor oil are available for specific purposes. For example, if you are looking for a skincare solution, a light and odorless castor oil may be preferable. For hair care, Jamaican Black Castor Oil is often recommended.

Read Customer Reviews

Gain insights from others who have used the product by reading customer reviews. Look for reviews from individuals with similar needs or concerns to yours to make a more informed decision.

Check for Certifications

Look for certifications such as USDA Organic or other relevant quality standards. These certifications ensure that the castor oil meets specific criteria for purity and production practices.

Price vs. Quality Balance

While price can be an indicator of quality, it's not always the case. Some high-quality castor oils are reasonably priced. Consider the overall value, taking into account factors like purity, extraction method, and certifications.

Conclusion

Choosing the right castor oil involves careful consideration of its type, purity, extraction method, and purpose. By following these tips, you can make an informed decision to ensure that you get the most out of this versatile and beneficial oil for your skincare, hair care, and overall well-being.

Conclusion

In concluding our exploration of the miraculous world of castor oil, it is evident that this unassuming elixir holds the key to unlocking numerous benefits for the body and soul. Throughout this journey, we've delved into the rich history, unraveled the science behind its magic, and uncovered the myriad ways in which castor oil can revolutionize your well-being.

One of the paramount revelations is castor oil's exceptional ability to nourish and fortify the skin, promoting a radiant and youthful complexion. Whether used as a soothing facial serum, a gentle makeup remover, or a hydrating body oil, the elixir's deep moisturizing properties rejuvenate and heal, leaving behind a glow that transcends mere aesthetics.

Our exploration also took us into the realm of hair care, where castor oil emerges as a potent tonic for lush and vibrant locks. From combating hair loss to stimulating growth, this elixir proves to be a versatile and indispensable asset in any beauty regimen. Its natural richness in nutrients ensures that your hair not only looks healthier but truly becomes healthier from root to tip.

Beyond its cosmetic allure, castor oil has demonstrated profound benefits for internal well-being. Its purgative qualities, when used judiciously, can aid in digestive health and detoxification. The elixir's anti-inflammatory properties further contribute to the maintenance of a resilient and robust immune system, offering a shield against various ailments.

As we conclude this journey, it is imperative to emphasize the simplicity with which castor oil can be seamlessly incorporated into your daily routine. Whether applied topically or ingested, its versatility allows for a myriad of applications, adapting effortlessly to your lifestyle. From the invigorating morning ritual of massaging a few drops onto your skin to the calming nighttime routine of adding it to your hair care regimen, the possibilities are as boundless as the benefits themselves.

In embracing the miracle elixir that is castor oil, you not only enhance your physical well-being but also connect with a time-honored tradition of natural healing. Let this book be your guide as you embark on a journey to unlock the secrets of castor oil, discovering the profound and transformative impact it can have on your life. May the elixir of castor oil continue to enrich your days, infusing them with health, beauty, and the timeless wisdom of nature.

References

Arslan, G. G., & Eşer, I. (2011). An examination of the effect of castor oil packs on constipation in the elderly. *Complementary therapies in clinical practice*, *17*(1), 58–62. https://doi.org/10.1016/j.ctcp.2010.04.004

Boddu, S. H., Alsaab, H., Umar, S., Bonam, S. P., Gupta, H., & Ahmed, S. (2015). Anti-inflammatory effects of a novel ricinoleic acid poloxamer gel system for transdermal delivery. *International journal of pharmaceutics*, *479*(1), 207–211. https://doi.org/10.1016/j.ijpharm.2014.12.051

Valera, M. C., Maekawa, L. E., de Oliveira, L. D., Jorge, A. O., Shygei, É., & Carvalho, C. A. (2013). In vitro antimicrobial activity of auxiliary chemical substances and natural extracts on Candida albicans and Enterococcus faecalis in root canals. *Journal of applied oral science: revista FOB*, *21*(2), 118–123. https://doi.org/10.1590/1678-7757201302135

Narayanan, S., Van Vleet, J., Strunk, B., Ross, R. N., & Gray, M. (2005). Comparison of pressure ulcer treatments in long-term care facilities: clinical outcomes and impact on cost. *Journal of wound, ostomy, and continence nursing: official publication of The Wound, Ostomy and Continence Nurses Society, 32*(3), 163–170. https://doi.org/10.1097/00152192-200505000-00004

Gavazzoni Dias M. F. (2015). Hair cosmetics: an overview. *International journal of trichology, 7*(1), 2–15. https://doi.org/10.4103/0974-7753.153450

Alookaran J, Tripp J. Castor Oil. [Updated 2022 Nov 21]. In: StatPearls [Internet]. Treasure Island (FL): StatPearls Publishing; 2024 Jan-. Available from: https://www.ncbi.nlm.nih.gov/books/NBK551626/

Arslan, G. G., & Eşer, I. (2011). An examination of the effect of castor oil packs on constipation in the elderly. *Complementary therapies in clinical practice, 17*(1), 58–62. https://doi.org/10.1016/j.ctcp.2010.04.004

Takashima, K., Komeda, Y., Sakurai, T., Masaki, S., Nagai, T., Matsui, S., Hagiwara, S., Takenaka, M., Nishida, N., Kashida, H., Nakaji, K., Watanabe, T., & Kudo, M. (2021). Castor oil as booster for colon capsule endoscopy preparation reduction: A prospective pilot study and patient questionnaire. *World journal of gastrointestinal pharmacology and therapeutics*, *12*(4), 79–89. https://doi.org/10.4292/wjgpt.v12.i4.79

Ghazikhanlou Sani, K., Jafari, M. R., & Shams, S. (2010). A comparison of the efficacy, adverse effects, and patient compliance of the sena-graph®syrup and castor oil regimens for bowel preparation. *Iranian journal of pharmaceutical research: IJPR*, *9*(2), 193–198.

Purnamawati, S., Indrastuti, N., Danarti, R., & Saefudin, T. (2017). The Role of Moisturizers in Addressing Various Kinds of Dermatitis: A Review. *Clinical medicine & research*, *15*(3-4), 75–87. https://doi.org/10.3121/cmr.2017.1363

Harwood A, Nassereddin A, Krishnamurthy K. Moisturizers. [Updated 2022 Aug 21]. In: StatPearls [Internet]. Treasure Island (FL): StatPearls Publishing; 2024 Jan-. Available from: https://www.ncbi.nlm.nih.gov/books/NBK545171/

Panico, A., Serio, F., Bagordo, F., Grassi, T., Idolo, A., DE Giorgi, M., Guido, M., Congedo, M., & DE Donno, A. (2019). Skin safety and health prevention:

an overview of chemicals in cosmetic products. *Journal of preventive medicine and hygiene*, *60*(1), E50–E57. https://doi.org/10.15167/2421-4248/jpmh2019.60.1.1080

Sánchez-Guerrero, I. M., Huertas, A. J., López, M. P., Carreño, A., Ramírez, M., & Pajarón, M. (2010). Angioedema-like allergic contact dermatitis to castor oil. *Contact dermatitis*, *62*(5), 318–319. https://doi.org/10.1111/j.1600-0536.2010.01733.x

Yalamanchili, P. S., Potluri, S., Surapaneni, H., Basha, M. H., & Davanapelly, P. (2016). Candidal Infection of the Gingiva Mimicking Desquamative Gingivitis: A Case Report. *Journal of clinical and diagnostic research: JCDR*, *10*(3), ZD04–ZD5. https://doi.org/10.7860/JCDR/2016/17413.7367

Hannah, V. E., O'Donnell, L., Robertson, D., & Ramage, G. (2017). Denture Stomatitis: Causes, Cures and Prevention. *Primary dental journal*, *6*(4), 46–51. https://doi.org/10.1308/205016817822230175

Pinelli, L. A., Montandon, A. A., Corbi, S. C., Moraes, T. A., & Fais, L. M. (2013). Ricinus communis treatment of denture stomatitis in institutionalised elderly. *Journal of oral rehabilitation*, *40*(5), 375–380. https://doi.org/10.1111/joor.12039

Salles, M. M., Badaró, M. M., Arruda, C. N., Leite, V. M., Silva, C. H., Watanabe, E., Oliveira, V.deC., & Paranhos, H.deF. (2015). Antimicrobial activity of complete denture cleanser solutions based on sodium hypochlorite and Ricinus communis - a randomized clinical study. *Journal of applied oral science: revista FOB*, *23*(6), 637–642. https://doi.org/10.1590/1678-775720150204